NCCN Guidelines for Patients®

The essential guide for people facing cancer.

Based on care recommendations from leading cancer experts.

Explains high-quality cancer care provided at state-of-the-art cancer centers.

Reviewed and revised every year.

Did you know that top cancer centers across the United States work together to improve cancer care? This alliance of leading cancer centers is called the National Comprehensive Cancer Network® (NCCN®).

Because cancer care is always evolving, NCCN develops and frequently updates evidence-based cancer care recommendations used by health care providers worldwide. These recommendations are known as the NCCN Clinical Practice Guidelines in Oncology (NCCN Guidelines®).

The NCCN Guidelines for Patients plainly explain these expert recommendations, so you can talk with your care team about the best care for you.

These NCCN Guidelines for Patients are based on the NCCN Guidelines® for B-Cell Lymphomas, Version 4.2026 — May 20, 2026.

View the NCCN Guidelines for Patients free online: NCCN.org/patientguidelines

Find an NCCN Cancer Center near you: NCCN.org/cancercenters

Learn how the NCCN Guidelines for Patients are developed: NCCN.org/patient-guidelines-process

Connect with us

@NCCNorg @NCCNVideo NCCN @NCCNorg

Supporters

NCCN Guidelines for Patients are supported by funding from the NCCN Foundation®

NCCN Foundation gratefully acknowledges the following corporate supporters for helping to make available these NCCN Guidelines for Patients: Lilly.

NCCN independently adapts, updates, and hosts the NCCN Guidelines for Patients. Our corporate supporters do not participate in the development of the NCCN Guidelines for Patients and are not responsible for the content and recommendations contained therein.

To make a gift, visit
NCCNFoundation.org/Donate

To learn more, visit online
NCCN.org/patientguidelines
or email
PatientGuidelines@NCCN.org

Contents

NCCN Foundation seeks to support the millions of patients and their families affected by a cancer diagnosis by funding and distributing NCCN Guidelines for Patients. NCCN Foundation is also committed to advancing cancer treatment by funding the nation's promising doctors at the center of innovation in cancer research. For more details and the full library of patient and caregiver resources, visit NCCN.org/patients.

National Comprehensive Cancer Network (NCCN) and NCCN Foundation
3025 Chemical Road, Suite 100, Plymouth Meeting, PA 19462 USA

1

About mantle cell lymphoma

Mantle cell lymphoma (MCL) is a rare but treatable cancer that starts in your body's immune system. It usually needs to be treated soon after it's diagnosed. But new treatments are giving people more hope and more years to live.

What is mantle cell lymphoma?

Mantle cell lymphoma (MCL) is a rare but treatable cancer that develops from certain white blood cells called lymphocytes. Lymphocytes normally protect the body from infection.

Cancer occurs when these cells multiply and grow out of control. An abnormal growth of lymphocytes is a form of cancer called lymphoma. Lymphoma usually affects the lymphatic system, but it can also affect other parts of the body.

What is the lymphatic system?

The lymphatic system is part of the immune (infection-fighting) system. It transports fluids to the bloodstream and fights germs.

The lymphatic system is made up of lymph fluid, lymph nodes, and other organs like the spleen. Lymph fluid contains infection-fighting lymphocytes. The lymphatic system is closely linked to the bloodstream and bone marrow, where new blood cells are made.

Lymph nodes (sometimes called "glands") are small, bean-shaped structures. Hundreds of lymph nodes are connected by lymph vessels throughout your body. Lymph nodes are usually clustered in groups in your neck, chest, armpits, groin, pelvis, and along your gut. The spleen, tonsils, and thymus are also part of the lymphatic system.

As lymph fluid travels through the body, lymph nodes catch and filter out foreign particles and harmful cells.

When you get an infection, an army of lymphocytes fills up your lymph nodes to fight it. That's why the lymph nodes in your neck feel swollen when you have a cold, flu, or sinus infection.

What is a mantle cell?

A mantle cell is a type of B cell inside lymph nodes.

Inside each lymph node are little round clumps of cells called follicles, which play a key role in the immune system.

Follicles contain mostly B cells, a type of lymphocyte that fights bacteria, viruses, and other pathogens. When a foreign substance enters the lymph node, these cells spring into action to break up the substance and get rid of it.

As part of this process, many follicle cells group together into a ball called the germinal center. Inside the germinal center, the cells attack the foreign substance.

Other follicle cells form a circle around the germinal center. This outer area is called the mantle zone. Mantle cell lymphoma starts in B cells in this region inside the lymph node.

What causes mantle cell lymphoma?

MCL occurs when lymphocytes develop a genetic change that causes them to start overproducing a protein called cyclin D1. This protein stimulates these altered cells to grow out of control and become lymphoma cells.

No one knows exactly what causes the mantle zone cells to develop this genetic change, but researchers are working on it.

MCL is different for everyone. For some people, it grows quickly over weeks to months. Such fast-growing lymphomas are described as aggressive. For other people, MCL grows slowly over years. Slow-growing MCL is watched closely for any changes.

People who have fast-growing MCL may receive different treatment from people with slow-growing MCL.

Where is the mantle zone?

The mantle zone is a ring of cells that surrounds the germinal center of a follicle (left). A follicle is a clump of cells inside a lymph node (center) where, normally, disease-fighting cells in the lymphatic system (right) attack harmful invaders.

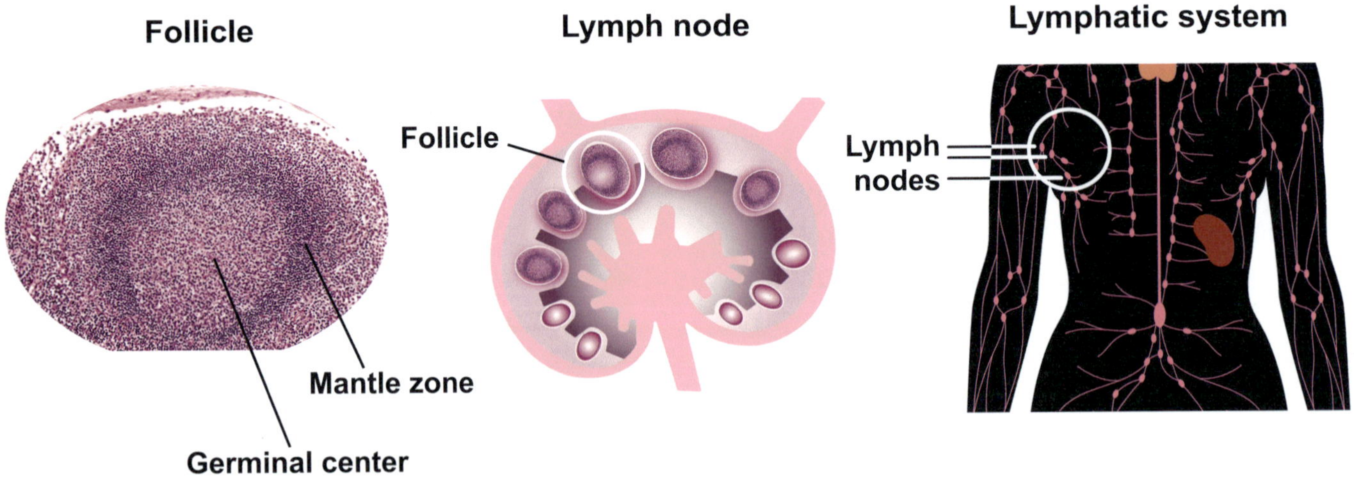

How is mantle cell lymphoma identified?

MCL is often discovered when a person has painless, swollen lymph nodes in the neck, armpit, or groin. The lymph nodes swell because of the overgrowth of lymphoma cells. Swollen lymph nodes are sometimes detected when an imaging test (like a CT scan) is done to look for the cause of a new symptom, or even for an unrelated reason.

Other MCL symptoms may include fever, drenching sweats at night, unexpected weight loss, fatigue, and stomach upset or pain.

Besides the lymph nodes, MCL is commonly found in the spleen, liver, bone marrow, blood stream, and gastrointestinal (GI) tract. The GI tract is made up of the stomach, intestines, and other organs that help digest food.

MCL is usually found in multiple parts of the body when it's first diagnosed. This is referred to as advanced-stage MCL. In rare cases, MCL may appear to be limited to a smaller (localized) area, which is called early-stage MCL. Early-stage MCL may be treated differently from advanced-stage MCL.

Multiple tests—like blood tests, genetic tests, and imaging scans—are needed to make sure it's MCL and not some other disease or type of lymphoma. These tests also find out how widespread the lymphoma is in the body.

Because MCL is a less common form of lymphoma, it can sometimes be difficult to diagnose and treat. If possible, seek out a medical center that specializes in lymphomas. You can also ask for a second opinion.

How is mantle cell lymphoma treated?

Treatment for MCL can include chemotherapy, immunotherapy, targeted therapy, radiation therapy, cellular therapy, or a combination of these treatments.

MCL is usually a lifelong disease. But treatment can slow its growth, reduce its symptoms, and prolong your life. For many people, treatment can put MCL into remission. Remission means there are no symptoms or signs of cancer. Remission may last for months or years. However, MCL may come back and need more or stronger treatment.

How can I get the best care?

Advocate for yourself. You have an important role to play in your care. Many people feel more satisfied when they actively take part in planning their cancer care.

The NCCN Guidelines for Patients will help you play a larger role in your care. Discuss the recommendations in this guide with your care team. Ask questions about your options and share your goals and concerns.

Don't know what to ask? You're not alone. That's why we include suggested questions to ask at the end of chapters.

Keep reading to find the best care for you.

How this guide can help you

Making decisions about lymphoma care is stressful. There's a lot to learn, and you don't know what the future holds.

Use this guide to get the information and support you need.

Patients, doctors, and other health care professionals trust the NCCN Guidelines for Patients. This guide uses clear, everyday language to explain current cancer care recommendations made by respected experts in the field. Their recommendations are based on the latest research and practices at leading cancer centers.

Your health is unique to you, so your lymphoma care should be, too. As you read this guide, you'll learn which treatments are likely to provide the best results for you. And you'll be better prepared to talk with your care team.

2

Testing for mantle cell lymphoma

A variety of tests are needed to find out if you have mantle cell lymphoma (MCL) and to determine which areas of the body it has affected. Tests are used to plan treatment and to check how well the treatment is working.

If you haven't already been diagnosed, this chapter will help you know what tests you may have and what to expect during testing. The exams and tests used to diagnose mantle cell lymphoma (MCL) are listed in **Guide 1**.

Bring someone with you to listen when you get test results, ask questions, and write down the answers.

Diagnosis vs. Prognosis

What's the difference between your diagnosis and your prognosis? These 2 words sound similar but they're quite different.

Diagnosis: The identification of an illness based on tests. The diagnosis names what illness you have.

Prognosis: The likely course and outcome of a disease. The prognosis predicts how your disease will turn out.

Health history

Your health care team needs to have all of your health information. They'll ask you about any health issues and treatments you've had.

Medical history

You'll be asked about any health challenges and treatments you've had during your lifetime. Be ready to talk about:

- Illnesses
- Injuries
- Health conditions
- Symptoms
- Medications and supplements

MCL can sometimes cause B symptoms. Let your care team know if you have any of these B symptoms:

- Fevers
- Heavy sweating at night
- Unexplained weight loss

MCL may also affect your gastrointestinal (GI) tract and bone marrow. The GI tract includes the mouth, stomach, intestines, and other organs involved in digestion. GI symptoms that may occur include diarrhea, bloody stools, blood loss you can't see (occult bleeding), and pain in your abdomen.

Family history

You'll also be asked about the health of relatives on both sides of your family. Be prepared to discuss any cancers or other health conditions in your close family members, especially your siblings, parents, and grandparents.

Physical exam

A physical exam of your body is done to look for signs of disease. It's also used to help assess what treatments may be options for you.

Checking for swelling

Certain parts of your body should be checked for swelling. Swelling of lymph nodes (lymphadenopathy) is often the first sign of MCL. Lymph nodes may be so swollen that they can be easily felt or seen under the skin. Your doctor will gently press on the areas of your body that have lymph nodes, such as your neck, armpits, and groin. Your doctor will also feel your spleen and liver to assess their size.

Your activity ability

Your health care team will also rate your overall health and ability to do basic daily activities like walking, cleaning, bathing, and so forth.

This is known as performance status. Doctors check your performance status for several reasons, one of which is to learn whether you can handle intense therapy.

Guide 1
Health exams and tests before lymphoma treatment

Health history and exams	• Medical history, including B symptoms • Physical exam, including lymph nodes, liver, and spleen • Ability to do daily activities (performance status)
Blood tests	• Complete blood count (CBC) with differential • Comprehensive metabolic panel • Lactate dehydrogenase (LDH) test • Uric acid
Infectious disease tests	• Hepatitis B test • Hepatitis C test
Imaging	• CT or PET/CT scans of chest, abdomen, pelvis (and neck, if needed) with contrast
Heart tests	• Echocardiogram or MUGA scan, if certain chemotherapy is planned
Biopsies	• Lymph node biopsy • Bone marrow aspiration and biopsy, if needed • Endoscopy or colonoscopy, if needed • Lumbar puncture, if needed

Blood tests

MCL can cause abnormal results on blood tests. These results are used to select treatment, anticipate prognosis, and monitor the progress and safety of therapy.

A blood test requires a sample of your blood. The sample is removed with a needle inserted into a vein. This is called a blood draw.

Tests of your blood sample include:

CBC with differential

A complete blood count (CBC) measures parts of the blood. Test results include measurements of white blood cells, red blood cells, and platelets. Lymphoma and other health conditions can cause low or high counts.

There are 5 types of white blood cells. A differential counts the number of each type of white blood cell. It also checks if the cell counts are in balance with each other.

Comprehensive metabolic panel

Your liver, bone, and other organs release chemicals into your blood. A comprehensive metabolic panel includes tests for up to 14 of these chemicals. The tests show if the levels of chemicals are too low or too high. Abnormal levels can be caused by lymphoma or other health conditions.

LDH test

High levels of the protein lactate dehydrogenase (LDH) can be caused by lymphoma or other health problems. If related to lymphoma, high levels of LDH may be a sign that treatment may be needed soon.

Swollen glands

Swelling of lymph nodes (such as the "glands" in your throat) is often one of the first signs of mantle cell lymphoma. Lymph nodes may be so swollen that they can be easily felt or seen under the skin. Your doctor will gently press on the areas of your body that have lymph nodes, such as your neck, armpits, and groin.

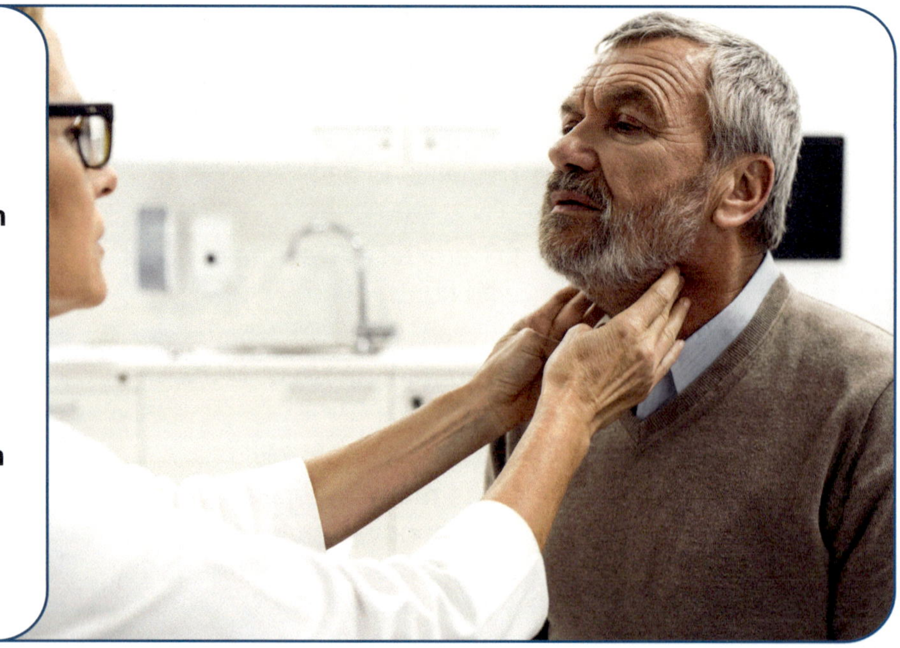

Uric acid

Uric acid is released by cells when DNA breaks down. You may have a high level of uric acid before starting treatment. Levels can be high due to fast-growing lymphoma, kidney disease, or other health conditions.

Hepatitis tests

Some types of lymphoma treatments can weaken your immune system. This increases your chance of getting infections. Hepatitis B and hepatitis C infections in particular can become active again from certain therapies. So it's important to be tested for hepatitis viruses.

Biopsies

The only way to be sure that you have lymphoma is to test fluid or tissue for lymphoma cells. A biopsy is a procedure that removes a sample of fluid or tissue for testing. There are several types of biopsies.

Lymph node biopsy

For B-cell lymphomas like MCL, experts from NCCN advise getting a biopsy that removes part or all of the lymph node through a cut into your skin.

However, a core needle biopsy may be necessary if the lymph node is difficult to get to. For a core needle biopsy, your clinician (usually an interventional radiologist) uses CT or ultrasound imaging to guide a long, hollow needle into the lymph node to obtain a sample of tissue.

Biopsy

A lymph node biopsy is a minor surgical procedure to remove a part or a whole lymph node. In this photo, the health care provider is using an ultrasound monitor to locate the area to be biopsied. After the procedure, the biopsy sample is tested to find out if it has lymphoma cells.

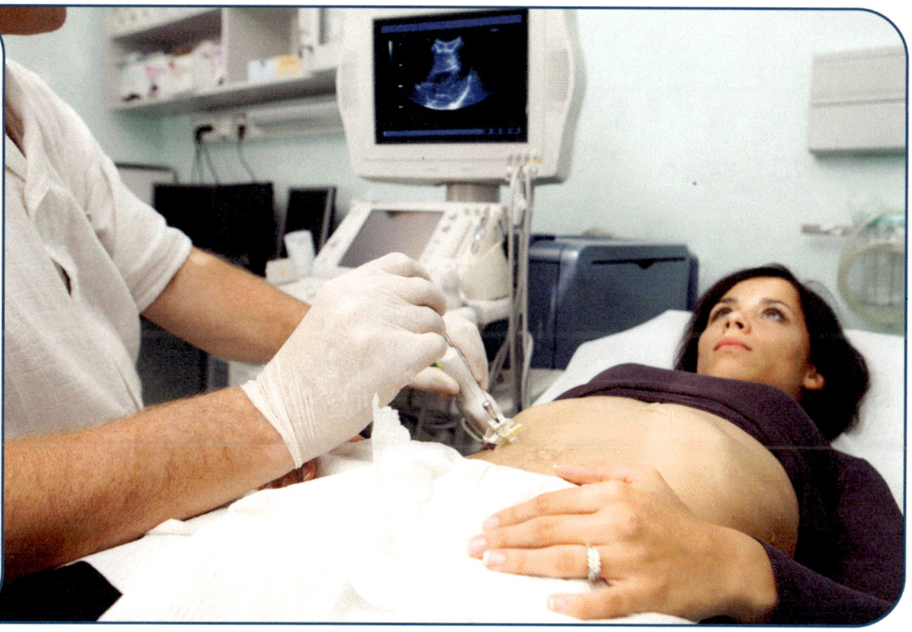

Bone marrow aspiration and biopsy

MCL can develop in bone marrow, which is part of the lymphatic system. A bone marrow biopsy removes a core of bone and soft bone marrow. A bone marrow aspiration removes liquid bone marrow. Both procedures may be done at the same time. The samples are sent to a lab for lymphoma testing.

GI biopsy

MCL is more likely than other types of lymphoma to involve the GI tract. To see inside the GI tract, doctors use procedures called endoscopy and colonoscopy. A device called an endoscope is used in the upper GI tract. A device called a colonoscope is used in the lower GI tract. Samples of tissue that may have lymphoma are removed and tested.

Lumbar puncture

A lumbar puncture is a procedure that removes a sample of spinal fluid. It's also called a spinal tap. Your doctor may suspect that the lymphoma is in spinal fluid based on symptoms or the lymphoma type.

Imaging

Imaging makes pictures of the insides of your body. It's used to detect lymphoma in deep lymph nodes, organs, bone marrow, and other parts of the body. It provides useful information to determine the extent of lymphoma involvement.

PET/CT

Positron emission tomography (PET) and computed tomography (CT or CAT scan) are 2 types of imaging. When used together, they're called a PET/CT scan. The PET/CT scan is used to image your whole body.

These tests are often used together to get the best picture before and after treatment.

PET scan

A PET scan requires injecting a substance called a radiotracer into your bloodstream. The radiotracer is detected with a special camera during the scan. It highlights cells that may be lymphoma. Afterward, the tracer leaves your body in your urine.

PET/CT scan

This is a PET/CT scanner. Imaging instruments, like this one, can detect even small amounts of lymphoma in your body.

During the scan, you lie down on a table that moves into the tunnel of the machine.

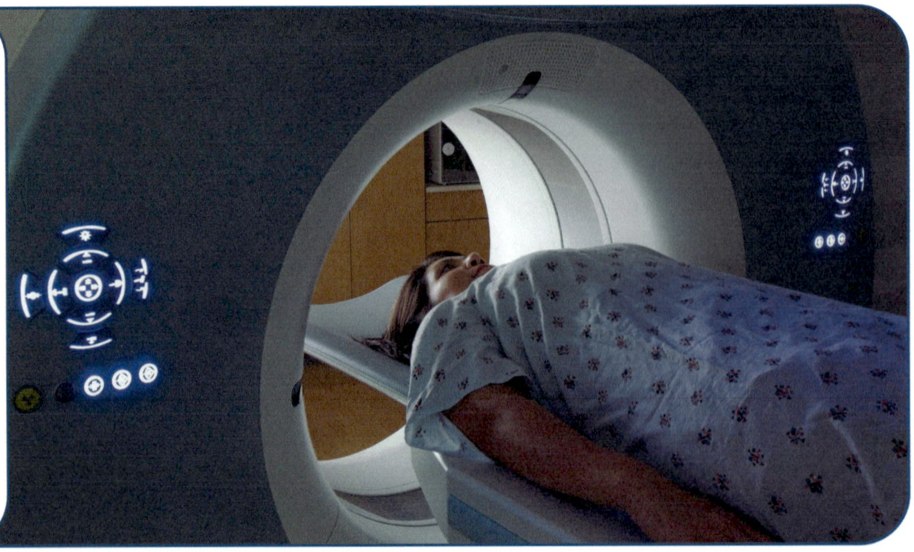

CT scan

A CT scan identifies lymph nodes and other tissues that may be enlarged. It uses x-rays to take many images from different angles. A computer then combines the pictures to make a series of cross-sectional images of your body.

A CT scan of your chest, belly area, and between your hip bones is needed to help diagnose MCL. You may also need a CT of your neck to look for lymphoma in lymph nodes.

Sometimes a contrast agent (also called contrast dye) is used to make the pictures clearer. Contrast is injected into the bloodstream and flushed out in urine.

Diagnostic tests

Cancers of blood cells, like MCL, can be difficult to tell apart. Diagnostic tests reveal which lymphoma you have.

For these tests, your blood and tissue samples are sent to a laboratory. At the lab, a doctor called a hematopathologist tests the samples to look for signs (markers) of MCL. Hematopathologists are experts at diagnosing lymphomas in blood cells.

Two tests they use are protein tests and molecular tests.

Protein tests

The hematopathologist will test your samples to look for proteins on the surface and inside of lymphoma cells. The hematopathologist looks for common patterns of proteins in the sample.

What is high-risk MCL?

High-risk MCL grows faster and may be more difficult to treat than typical MCL.

Three important, but uncommon, characteristics are associated with high-risk MCL:

- A high level of Ki-67 protein in lymphoma cells
- Lymphoma cells that divide rapidly and have an immature-looking (blastoid) cell appearance
- A mutation in the *TP53* gene

Treatments are available, but experts strongly recommend that people with high-risk MCL try to enroll in a clinical trial, if possible.

Finding, or not finding, these proteins can reveal the type of lymphoma. For example, MCL cells have high levels of a protein called cyclin D1, as well as CD5, CD20, SOX11, and other specific proteins.

At the same time, the proteins CD200 and LEF1 are usually missing in MCL. So a sample that contains the first group of proteins but doesn't contain the second group of proteins suggests a diagnosis of MCL.

Protein tests are important for diagnosing MCL. They can also give an idea of how quickly the MCL is growing. For example, some types of MCL don't produce the SOX11 protein, which may indicate a slow-growing MCL.

Ki-67 is another protein that's meaningful for MCL. High levels of Ki-67 show that the MCL is growing quickly.

The hematopathologist will also look at your cells under a microscope to find any visible abnormalities.

For instance, large, very rapidly dividing cells may indicate a rare subtype of MCL called blastoid variant. This subtype may be seen at diagnosis or appear later on. Blastoid-variant MCL grows faster and is more difficult to treat than typical MCL.

Molecular biomarker tests

Genes and chromosomes contain the instructions to make cells work and to make new cells. Abnormal changes in genes and chromosomes can lead to lymphoma. Sometimes it helps to test for these changes. The results can be used for diagnosis and prognosis.

Most MCL cells are known to have a specific change, called a translocation, in their chromosomes. A translocation means that 2 chromosomes have switched specific parts.

The MCL translocation occurs when a part of chromosome 14 trades places with a part of chromosome 11. This translocation is what causes cells to make too much cyclin D1, a protein that helps control cell replication. Too much of this protein leads to the development of MCL.

Translocation

Translocation means that parts of 2 chromosomes are switched.

The translocation in mantle cell lymphoma occurs when the bottom of chromosome 11 switches places with the bottom of chromosome 14. This leads to an increase in cyclin D1, a protein that helps control the cell cycle.

The presence of too much cyclin D1 is one of the key features of MCL.

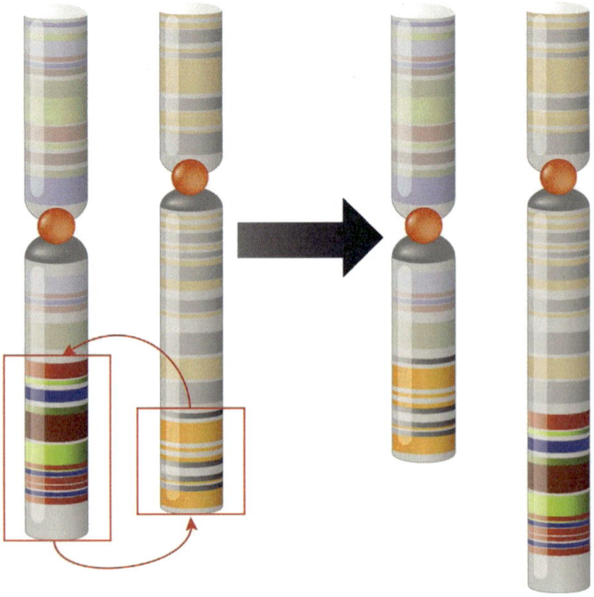

Using biopsy samples, the hematopathologist can test the chromosomes in your cells to find out if they have this genetic abnormality.

MCL also involves other changes. Certain abnormal changes in genes can affect how well the lymphoma is likely to respond to treatment. So it may be useful to test for certain genes that have abnormal changes.

In particular, an abnormal change (mutation) in the *TP53* gene is linked to faster-growing MCL and poor results with standard lymphoma treatment. So anyone with MCL should consider genetic testing of their biopsy sample to check the *TP53* gene.

Also ask about testing for other gene mutations, which could help choose treatment and follow the lymphoma over time.

Heart tests

Some lymphoma treatments can damage your heart. To plan treatment, your doctor may test how well your heart pumps blood.

You may get an echocardiogram or multigated acquisition (MUGA) scan. An echocardiogram uses sound waves to make pictures of your heart. A MUGA scan makes pictures using a tracer and special camera.

Fertility and pregnancy

Some lymphoma treatments may affect your ability to conceive or bear children. However, options are available. Sperm can be frozen and stored in a sperm bank until after lymphoma treatment. Eggs can be removed from ovaries and stored for later use. Discuss your thoughts and preferences with your health care team.

Some lymphoma treatments can harm an unborn baby. If you could be pregnant, expect to take a pregnancy test before you start treatment. Also, take steps to avoid getting pregnant or causing a pregnancy during treatment. Your care team can tell you which birth control methods are best to use.

Key points

- Your health care team will check the size of your lymph nodes, spleen, and liver.
- Blood tests will be done to look for signs of lymphoma and other health issues.
- A biopsy or special testing is the only way to be sure that you have mantle cell lymphoma (MCL). Lymph nodes and other areas of your body may also need to be biopsied.
- Imaging tests like CT and PET scans allow your care providers to look inside your body to find where the lymphoma is located.
- Protein tests identify a signature-like pattern of proteins that can reveal whether you have MCL or another type of lymphoma.
- Molecular tests can find certain genetic changes that may confirm the diagnosis and help understand your prognosis.

Questions to ask

- Where do I go to get tested? How long will the tests take? Will any of the tests hurt?
- Will my insurance pay for all of the tests you're recommending?
- How soon will I know the results and who will explain them to me?
- Who will talk with me about the next steps? When?
- Is my MCL high-risk? How quickly is it growing?

"Try to remember that everyone's journey is different. Your physiological, mental, emotional, and spiritual response is unique."

3
Types of treatment

There isn't one single recommended treatment for mantle cell lymphoma (MCL)—there are many treatment options. You and your health care team will work together to figure out the best treatment for you.

Treatment decisions are based on different factors such as your age, level of fitness (performance status), and overall health. Often the most important factor is the extent of the lymphoma. Doctors classify this by cancer stage.

Cancer stage

A cancer stage is a number that stands for how much cancer is in the body and where it's located. For mantle cell lymphoma (MCL), the stage represents how many areas of the body are affected by lymphoma. Fewer areas of lymphoma in the body equal a lower stage number, and more areas of lymphoma equal a higher stage number. This number is based mostly on the results of your biopsies, blood tests, and imaging.

Doctors use a specific rating system for most lymphomas. This system includes 4 stages. For treatment purposes, the stages are often grouped together like this:

Stage 1 and stage 2 refer to early-stage (localized) MCL. These lymphomas haven't progressed to many locations in the body. MCL is rarely diagnosed at these stages. For more information about stage 1 and stage 2 MCL, see *Chapter 5: Treatment for early mantle cell lymphoma*.

Stage 3 and stage 4 represent advanced-stage MCL. In these stages, the lymphoma occurs in lymph nodes in several areas in the body. It may also be found in the spleen, bone marrow, or other organs. Almost all people with MCL are diagnosed when the lymphoma has reached these stages.

Treatment options for advanced-stage MCL are partly based on how fast the lymphoma is growing. Advanced-stage MCL is described as fast growing or slow growing. Most people who are diagnosed with advanced-stage MCL have the fast-growing kind.

Treatment types

Treating MCL includes treatment of the lymphoma and support for you.

The aim of treatment is to reduce symptoms, control the cancer, get the lymphoma into remission, and extend life. Remission means that the lymphoma can't be detected.

Researchers are always testing new treatments. Newer treatments are helping people with MCL live longer with fewer health challenges than before. While MCL can be thought of as an ongoing (chronic) disease, a number of people now achieve long-lasting remission after treatment.

Not everyone receives the same treatment, though. Also, some people can handle more intense treatment while others cannot. Your doctor will tailor your treatment based on the tests described in *Chapter 2: Testing for MCL*.

Why some therapies are preferred

All treatments listed in this guide are recommended and appropriate. When helpful, NCCN experts also assign a level of preference to their recommendations for systemic therapies. Their recommendations are grouped into 3 categories:

Preferred therapies have the most evidence they may work better and be safer than other therapies.

Other recommended therapies can provide effective results but may have less evidence, more side effects, or may not work quite as well as preferred therapies.

Therapies used in certain cases work best for individuals with specific lymphoma features or health circumstances.

Current types of treatment for MCL include chemoimmunotherapy, targeted therapy, and other types of therapy.

Chemoimmunotherapy

This treatment combines the use of chemotherapy and immunotherapy. It's one of the most potent treatment options for MCL.

Chemotherapy uses drugs to damage and destroy rapidly dividing cells, like lymphoma cells. Chemotherapy harms healthy cells, too. That's why it can cause side effects. Some chemotherapy drugs are given through an intravenous (IV) infusion into a vein in your arm or another part of your body. Other types of chemotherapy can be taken as a pill.

Chemotherapy is given in treatment cycles. One cycle is made up of a few days of treatment followed by a period of rest. This lets the body recover before the next cycle. One cycle is often 3 or 4 weeks long. However, the cycle schedule varies depending on which drugs are used.

Chemoimmunotherapy

Chemoimmunotherapy combines chemotherapy and immunotherapy treatments. These treatments used together are often more effective than both treatments used separately.

Some chemotherapy drugs are given through an intravenous (IV) infusion into a vein in your arm. This patient is receiving chemotherapy through an IV access port in the upper chest.

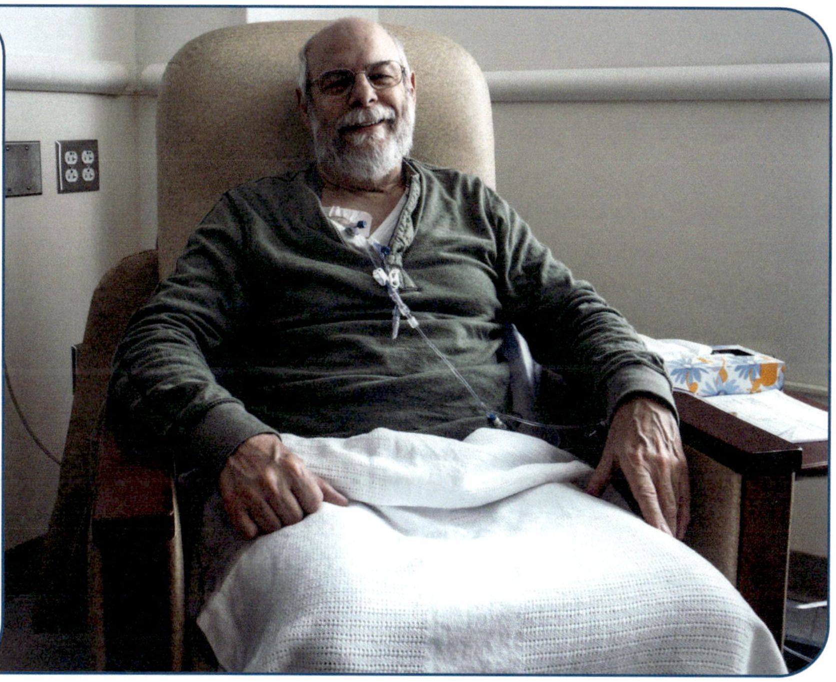

What is a regimen?

A regimen is a plan that defines the dosage, schedule, and duration of a treatment. Regimens for MCL often include multiple drugs.

Immunotherapy consists of medicines that are based on antibodies. Antibodies are natural proteins of the immune system. They help your body fight germs and other threats.

Antibodies can also be made in a lab. These antibodies are designed to treat specific types of lymphoma. Rituximab (Rituxan) is a monoclonal antibody treatment for MCL. It recognizes and attaches to a specific protein (CD20) that's found on the surface of most B cells. Rituximab marks these cells so that your immune system can find and destroy them. Rituximab is given through an IV.

For chemoimmunotherapy, some regimens are intense and some are less intense. Good results can be achieved with both types of regimens. Intense regimens have more risk of side effects, so they aren't often given to older adults or those with other health conditions.

Targeted therapy

Targeted therapy drugs attack certain molecules in lymphoma cells to halt their growth and spread. Targeted therapy harms normal cells less than chemotherapy does.

Types of targeted therapies for MCL include:

Kinase inhibitors – Kinases are enzymes with many cell functions. A kinase called Bruton's tyrosine kinase (BTK) helps cancerous B cells develop and grow. Drugs that block BTK can reduce the number of new MCL cells that are made. These drugs, called BTK inhibitors, include acalabrutinib (Calquence), ibrutinib (Imbruvica), pirtobrutinib (Jaypirca), and zanubrutinib (Brukinsa). BTK inhibitors are oral medicines given as capsules or tablets.

BCL-2 inhibitors – BCL-2 is a protein inside of B cells that helps prevent cell death. BCL-2 can build up in lymphoma cells and save them from dying. BCL-2 inhibitors are drugs that block the effect of BCL-2. This allows the lymphoma cells to self-destruct. BCL-2 inhibitors, which include venetoclax (Venclexta) and sonrotoclax (Beqalzi), are given as tablets. They're currently used only for advance-stage MCL after having other regimens.

Proteasome inhibitors – Bortezomib (Velcade) is a drug that targets proteasomes inside lymphoma cells. Proteasomes are sometimes called the cell's "garbage disposal" because they grind up and get rid of the cell's waste. Bortezomib halts the proteasomes from working. This causes waste to pile up in the lymphoma cell, which can poison and kill it. Bortezomib is given through an IV into a vein or under the skin.

Bispecific antibodies – A bispecific antibody is a drug that targets 2 different types of cells at the same time. For MCL, the 2 cell types are B cells, which can become cancerous, and T cells, which are immune cells that fight cancer cells. When the bispecific antibody binds to one of each cell, the T cell attacks and destroys the adjacent B cell.

Bispecific antibodies that treat MCL include glofitamab-gxbm (Columvi) and mosunetuzumab-axgb (Lunsumio). For MCL treatment, mosunetuzumab-axgb may be combined with polatuzumab vedotin-piiq (Polivy), which is a different type of drug called an antibody-drug conjugate. It also targets cancerous B cells. Bispecific antibodies are currently used to treat certain advanced cases of MCL.

Immunomodulators

Immunomodulators are drugs that are used in lymphoma care to boost the immune system. Lenalidomide (Revlimid) is an immunomodulator that's used to treat MCL. It's given as a capsule. Lenalidomide is usually given with rituximab.

Radiation therapy

Radiation therapy uses high-energy x-rays to treat MCL. The x-rays damage the DNA in lymphoma cells. This either kills the lymphoma cells or stops new lymphoma cells from being made.

A very focused type of radiation, involved-site radiation therapy (ISRT), is used for MCL that's confined to a limited area. ISRT targets only the lymphoma in the lymph node or affected area while avoiding the surrounding areas. This reduces many of the side effects of regular radiation therapy.

Radiation therapy may also be used for certain cases of MCL that come back after treatment (relapse).

Stem cell transplant

A stem cell transplant aims to extend the improvement you receive from your current treatment and to prolong your life.

But it's an intense treatment. Stem cell transplant is now used only in certain cases for treating MCL. So it may not be part of your care plan.

There are 2 types of stem cell transplants:

An autologous transplant is also called high-dose therapy with autologous stem cell rescue (or HDT/ASCR). First, many of your healthy stem cells will be removed and stored for later. Next, you'll receive high doses of chemotherapy to destroy the lymphoma cells. Chemotherapy will also wipe out the blood-producing cells in the bone marrow. Your healthy stem cells will then be returned to your body to "rescue" your bone marrow.

An allogeneic transplant uses healthy stem cells from a donor. You'll first receive treatment, called conditioning, to help prevent your body from rejecting the transplanted cells. Next, you'll receive the donor cells, which will form new, healthy bone marrow and a new immune system. The new immune system will then attack lymphoma cells that weren't killed by earlier treatment.

CAR T-cell therapy

This treatment may be used if chemoimmunotherapy and targeted therapy aren't enough to halt the lymphoma. Chimeric antigen receptor (CAR) T-cell therapy is a treatment made from your own T cells. T cells are lymphocytes that hunt and destroy lymphoma cells, infected cells, and other damaged cells.

However, lymphoma cells learn how to hide from your T cells, which allows the lymphoma to grow. CAR T-cell therapy reprograms your natural T cells to recognize and attack lymphoma cells.

First, your own T cells are removed from your body using a special machine. At a lab, a CAR gene is added to your T cells. This genetically alters the T cells to hunt specifically for lymphoma cells. The CAR T cells are then infused back into your body where they find and kill MCL cells.

Two CAR-T therapies are currently used to treat certain cases of relapsed or refractory MCL. These are brexucabtagene autoleucel (Tecartus) and lisocabtagene maraleucel (Breyanzi).

Active surveillance

In some cases, no treatment is the right treatment. This may be the case with slow-growing MCL that isn't causing any symptoms.

While treatment may not be necessary, having regular tests and visits is still recommended to see if the lymphoma begins to grow. This is why it's called active surveillance. (It's also called watch-and-wait.) If symptoms begin, treatment will also begin.

Clinical trials

Another potential way to get treatment MCL is by joining a clinical trial.

A clinical trial is a type of medical research study. After being developed and tested in a lab, potential new ways of fighting cancer need to be studied in people.

If found to be safe and effective in a clinical trial, a drug, device, or treatment approach may be approved by the U.S. FDA.

Everyone with cancer should carefully consider all of the treatment options available for their cancer type, including standard treatments and clinical trials. Talk to your doctor about whether a clinical trial may make sense for you.

Phases

Most cancer clinical trials focus on treatment and are done in phases.

- **Phase 1** trials study the safety and side effects of an investigational drug or treatment approach.
- **Phase 2** trials study how well the drug or approach works against a specific type of cancer.
- **Phase 3** trials test the drug or approach against a standard treatment. If the results are good, it may be approved by the FDA.
- **Phase 4** trials study the safety and benefit of an FDA-approved treatment.

Who can enroll?

It depends on the clinical trial's rules, called eligibility criteria. The rules may be about age, cancer type and stage, treatment history, or general health. They ensure that participants are alike in specific ways and that the trial is as safe as possible for the participants.

Informed consent

Clinical trials are managed by a research team. This group of experts will review the study with you in detail, including its purpose and the risks and benefits of joining. All of this information is also provided in an informed consent form. Read the form carefully and ask questions before signing it. Take time to discuss it with people you trust. Keep in mind that you can leave and seek treatment outside of the clinical trial at any time.

Will I get a placebo?

Placebos (inactive versions of real medicines) are almost never used alone in cancer clinical trials. It is common to receive either a placebo with a standard treatment, or a new drug with a standard treatment. You will be informed, verbally and in writing, if a placebo is part of a clinical trial before you enroll.

Are clinical trials free?

There is no fee to enroll in a clinical trial. The study sponsor pays for research-related costs, including the study drug. But you may need to pay for other services, like transportation or childcare, due to extra appointments. During the trial, you will continue to receive standard cancer care. This care is often covered by insurance.

Finding a clinical trial

In the United States

NCCN Cancer Centers
NCCN.org/cancercenters

The National Cancer Institute (NCI)
cancer.gov/about-cancer/treatment/clinical-trials/search

Worldwide

The U.S. National Library of Medicine (NLM)
clinicaltrials.gov

Need help finding a clinical trial?

NCI's Cancer Information Service (CIS)
1.800.4.CANCER (1.800.422.6237)
cancer.gov/contact

Treatment for side effects

All treatments can cause unwanted health problems called side effects. Some side effects may be harmful to your health. Others may just be unpleasant.

Different treatments have different side effects. Side effects also depend on the length or dose of treatment and the person.

Most side effects appear shortly after treatment starts and go away in days or weeks after treatment is over. Other side effects may be long-term or appear years later.

Don't ignore or disregard side effects. If left untreated, they may delay your scheduled treatment. Tell your health care team about any new or worse symptoms you have.

Ask your treatment team for a complete list of the side effects of your treatments. There are ways to prevent some side effects and help you feel better.

"Ask your oncologist for a list of possible side effects right before each treatment. Track your side effects and report them to your doctor.

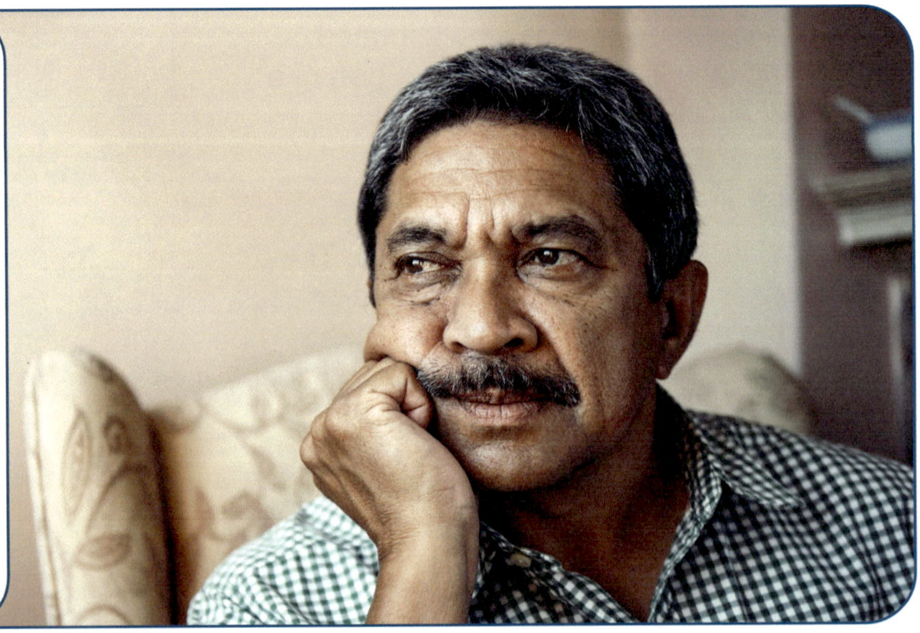

Supportive care

Supportive care helps improve your quality of life during and after lymphoma treatment. The goal is to prevent or manage side effects and symptoms, like pain and fatigue.

Supportive care (also called palliative care) is available to everyone with MCL and their families, not just those at the end of life. In fact, people who start supportive care when they begin treatment tend to have improved outcomes and better quality of life.

Read more about supportive care in *Chapter 6: Treatment for recurrent MCL*.

"A common myth is that palliative care is only for terminally ill patients. It is so much more! Palliative care providers treat the whole patient, not just cancer. It's worth reaching out to Palliative Care in your hospital or clinic."

Common side effects of MCL treatments

- Tiredness
- Nausea
- Vomiting
- Diarrhea
- Headache
- Low blood cell counts
- Constipation
- Infection
- Fever or chills
- Decreased appetite
- Rash
- Sores and swelling in the mouth
- Shortness of breath
- Heart problems
- Hair loss
- Tingling, numbness, or pain in hands or feet

Key points

- Often the most important factor for deciding on treatment is the extent of the lymphoma—how many areas of the body it has affected.
- Stage 1 and stage 2 refer to early-stage mantle cell lymphoma (MCL). MCL is rarely diagnosed in its early stages.
- Stage 3 and stage 4 represent advanced-stage MCL. Almost all people with MCL are diagnosed when the lymphoma has reached an advanced stage.
- Chemotherapy uses drugs to kill lymphoma cells. Immunotherapy uses manufactured antibodies to destroy lymphoma cells. Chemoimmunotherapy is a more effective combination of these 2 treatments.
- Targeted therapy drugs attack certain molecules in lymphoma cells to halt their growth and spread.
- Clinical trials study the safety and effectiveness of an investigational drug or treatment approach.
- All treatments cause side effects. Be sure to tell your treatment team if you get any physical or emotional effects after treatment.

Questions to ask

- What are my treatment options?
- What are the benefits and risks of each treatment option?
- Are you suggesting treatment options from the NCCN Guidelines, or have you modified the standard approach for my situation?
- Will the treatment hurt or cause a lot of side effects?
- How do I get a second opinion?

4

Treatment for advanced mantle cell lymphoma

Most people diagnosed with mantle cell lymphoma (MCL) have advanced disease. Advanced-stage MCL requires multi-drug therapy, but treatment methods continue to evolve. This chapter explains the treatment process.

People who have stage 3 or stage 4 mantle cell lymphoma (MCL) are considered to have **advanced-stage MCL**. (For information about early-stage MCL, see *Chapter 5: Treatment for early mantle cell lymphoma*.)

The goal of treating advanced MCL is to remove as much lymphoma as possible and keep the disease under control. Treatment may continue for months or even years.

Treatment for advanced-stage MCL depends on whether the lymphoma is growing fast or growing slow.

Most people diagnosed with advanced-stage MCL have the fast-growing type. Read the next section to learn about treatment for fast-growing MCL. (For treatment for slow-growing MCL, see page 36.)

First-line therapy has 2 to 3 steps

Primary treatment

reduces the amount of lymphoma as much as possible

↓

Additional treatment

(if needed) reinforces the results of primary treatment and delays the lymphoma from coming back

↓

Maintenance treatment

keeps the lymphoma under control or prevents it from coming back

Treatment for fast-growing MCL

One highly recommended option for fast-growing advanced-stage MCL is to receive treatment through an appropriate clinical trial.

But if you don't want to enroll in a clinical trial or if no trials are available, then you'll likely need more than one type of therapy for fast-growing advanced-stage MCL.

The first therapy you're given—called first-line therapy—is the one with the greatest likelihood to work.

However, if the lymphoma comes back after first-line therapy, further treatment is available. Your next therapy is called second-line therapy.

If the lymphoma comes back after both first-line and second-line therapy, you may want to try a third-line therapy.

First-line therapy

First-line therapy is given in 2 or 3 phases: primary treatment, additional treatment (if needed), and maintenance treatment.

Primary treatment

The goal of primary treatment is to reduce the amount of lymphoma as much as possible. The choice of treatment depends on whether or not your body can handle intense (aggressive) therapy. Preferred primary treatments are listed in **Guide 3**.

If your body can't handle aggressive treatment, see the preferred options for moderate treatment in **Guide 4**.

What is a relapse?

Although newer approaches to treatment have improved results, most people with MCL eventually have a relapse.

A relapse is when lymphoma gets better after treatment but later returns.

Relapse occurs because most drugs eventually begin to lose their effectiveness against the lymphoma. In other words, the lymphoma becomes resistant to the drug.

Each time MCL relapses, it may be more difficult to treat than the time before.

Your primary treatment will be a combination of different therapies. Doctors often use abbreviations to make it simpler to talk about these combinations. But people taking these regimens may find these abbreviations confusing. To decode the abbreviations, see **Guide 2**.

After primary treatment, your doctor will evaluate the results to see how well the therapy worked:

Complete response – If the usual tests can no longer detect the lymphoma, you've had a complete response to primary treatment. A complete response is also called remission. The lymphoma can still return, but you can stop primary treatment and begin maintenance treatment.

Guide 2
What do these treatment abbreviations mean?

ABR	**A**calabrutinib, **B**endamustine, **R**ituximab
AR	**A**calabrutinib, **R**ituximab
BR	**B**endamustine, **R**ituximab
CHOP plus Rituximab (RCHOP)	**C**yclophosphamide, Doxorubicin (**H**ydroxydaunorubicin), Vincristine (**O**ncovin), **P**rednisone plus **R**ituximab • Doxorubicin is also called Hydroxydaunorubicin • Oncovin is a brand name for Vincristine
DHA	**D**examethasone, **H**igh-Dose Cytarabine (**A**ra-C) • Ara-C stands for Cytosine Arabinoside, also called Cytarabine
GEMOX	**Gem**citabine, **Ox**aliplatin
IR	**I**brutinib, **R**ituximab
LR	**L**enalidomide, **R**ituximab
RBAC	**R**ituximab, **B**endamustine, Low-Dose Cytarabine (**A**ra-**C**)
RDHAP	**R**ituximab, **D**examethasone, **H**igh-Dose Cytarabine (**A**ra-C), **P**latinum-based chemotherapy
VR-CAP	Bortezomib (**V**elcade), **R**ituximab, **C**yclophosphamide, Doxorubicin (**A**driamycin), **P**rednisone • Velcade is a brand name for Bortezomib • Adriamycin is a brand name for Doxorubicin

Partial response – A partial response to primary treatment means that the lymphoma has decreased in size but is still there. If you have a partial response, you may need additional treatment.

No response – If the lymphoma continues to grow or seems unaffected by first-line therapy, you can have additional lines of therapy. See *Chapter 6: Treatment for recurrent MCL*.

Additional treatment

Additional treatment builds upon primary treatment to delay the lymphoma from coming back for as long as possible.

This additional treatment comes before maintenance treatment.

Which type of additional treatment you'll get depends on very sensitive lab tests that look for minimal residual disease (MRD). MRD means that there's still a tiny trace of lymphoma cells—an amount that's too small to be found by usual testing.

Guide 3
Aggressive primary treatments for advanced MCL (in alphabetical order)

Preferred treatments	**BR/RC**	(Bendamustine plus Rituximab) followed by High-Dose Cytarabine plus Rituximab
	LYMA regimen	DHA (Dexamethasone, High-Dose Cytarabine) and platinum-based chemotherapy plus Rituximab, followed by CHOP (Cyclophosphamide, Doxorubicin, Vincristine, Prednisone) plus Rituximab
	NORDIC regimen	Dose-intensified immunochemotherapy with CHOP plus Rituximab, alternating with High-Dose Cytarabine plus Rituximab
	TRIANGLE regimen	CHOP, a BTK inhibitor, plus Rituximab, alternating with DHA and platinum-based chemotherapy plus Rituximab
Other recommended treatment	**RBAC**	(Bendamustine, Low-Dose Cytarabine) plus Rituximab

If your lab tests find minimal residual disease after your primary treatment, then you might have additional treatment with HDT/ASCR (high-dose chemotherapy followed by an autologous stem cell rescue) to eliminate it—with the goal of achieving a long remission.

However, the use of HDT/ASCR is currently changing because it uses very high doses of chemotherapy and is relatively risky.

If the lab tests **don't** find any MRD, or if your doctor doesn't recommend HDT/ASCR for you, then you'll skip additional treatment and start maintenance treatment right after your primary treatment.

If you didn't achieve a complete response to primary treatment, then you could have additional treatment to try to get the lymphoma into remission.

If you haven't been treated with a BTK inhibitor before, then the preferred additional treatment in this case is targeted therapy with a BTK inhibitor.

A different chemoimmunotherapy regimen could be another treatment option that might provide a complete response.

Guide 4
Less aggressive primary treatments for advanced MCL (in alphabetical order)

Preferred treatments	**ABR**	Acalabrutinib, Bendamustine, plus Rituximab
	AR	Acalabrutinib plus Rituximab
	BR	Bendamustine plus Rituximab
Other recommended treatments	**CHOP plus Rituximab**	(Cyclophosphamide, Doxorubicin, Vincristine, Prednisone) plus Rituximab
	IR	Ibrutinib plus Rituximab
	LR	Lenalidomide plus Rituximab
	VR-CAP	(Bortezomib, Cyclophosphamide, Doxorubicin, Prednisone) plus Rituximab

Maintenance treatment

The goal of maintenance treatment is to prevent or delay the lymphoma from coming back. Or, if the lymphoma is still present, maintenance treatment may keep it under control.

Maintenance treatment typically includes rituximab given by intravenous (IV) infusion every 8 weeks for up to 2 to 3 years.

Your maintenance treatment may also include a BTK inhibitor, which can be given for 2 years or longer. This treatment may depend on your individual case, including your age, the type of primary therapy you had and your response to it, and the risk of side effects from a BTK inhibitor.

Follow-up care

During the maintenance phase, you'll have follow-up visits every few months with your doctor and care team. You'll also be tested for any signs that MCL has returned (relapsed) and be checked for any side effects. If you continue to have no signs of lymphoma, you'll have fewer follow-up visits over time.

If you have a relapse or recurrence, you can ask your care team to help you find a clinical trial. If you can't find a suitable clinical trial, you can move on to second-line treatment. For information on second-line treatment, see *Chapter 6: Treatment for recurrent mantle cell lymphoma*.

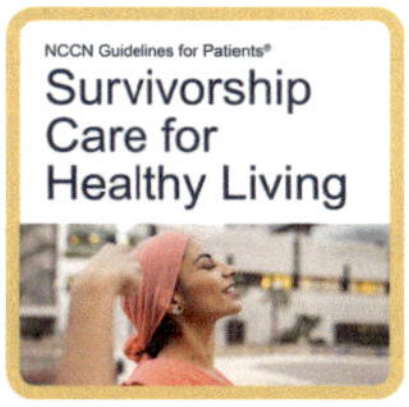

Survivorship

Living with cancer is called survivorship. It starts when your lymphoma is diagnosed.

Read more about survivorship in *NCCN Guidelines for Patients: Survivorship Care for Healthy Living*, available at NCCN.org/patientguidelines and on the NCCN Patient Guides for Cancer app.

"Report any unusual feelings of sadness, loss of interest in activities, anxiety, and sleep problems to your doctor. Many people experience these feelings, and they should not go untreated."

Treatment for slow-growing MCL

People with slow-growing MCL often have no symptoms and no swollen glands when they're diagnosed. The lymphoma occurs only in their bone marrow and blood (although some individuals may have it in their spleen or gastrointestinal tract).

Slow-growing MCL can exist for months, or even years, before it needs to be treated.

For people with slow-growing MCL that has no symptoms, doctors often take a watch-and-wait approach instead of starting treatment immediately. Watch-and-wait, also called active surveillance, means you'll have no treatment, but you'll continue to have tests to check for any signs of lymphoma.

If you begin to have MCL symptoms, you'll need to be re-evaluated. This may include another biopsy and also repeating some advanced testing on the biopsy sample.

Treatment for MCL with a *TP53* mutation

If molecular biomarker testing found that your lymphoma has a change in the *TP53* gene, NCCN experts strongly recommend participating in a clinical trial as an initial treatment option.

If you don't want to try to enroll in a clinical trial or no clinical trials are available, another treatment option is a combination of obinutuzumab (Gazyva), venetoclax (Venclexta), and zanubrutinib (Brukinsa).

Otherwise, treatment depends on whether or not your body can handle aggressive therapy.

Aggressive therapy – If you can undergo aggressive therapy, the recommended first treatment is the TRIANGLE regimen, which is described in **Guide 3**. This regimen is followed by maintenance therapy with rituximab infusion every 8 weeks for 3 years as well as a daily BTK inhibitor (acalabrutinib, ibrutinib, or zanubrutinib) for 2 years, or until the lymphoma returns.

Less aggressive therapy – If your care team recommends less aggressive first-line therapy, the suggested primary treatment is a BTK inhibitor (acalabrutinib) plus rituximab.

If your lymphoma returns, turn to *Chapter 6: Treatment for recurrent MCL*.

If you develop symptoms or have other signs that the lymphoma is growing, then you and your doctor should decide whether treatment should begin. To find out about treatment, see "Treatment for fast-growing MCL" on page 31.

Key points

- The goal of treatment is to remove as much of the lymphoma as possible and keep the disease under control.
- First-line treatment is often given in phases. The first phase is primary therapy. The most common primary therapy for advanced-stage MCL is chemoimmunotherapy with or without a BTK inhibitor.
- Primary treatment may be followed by additional treatment, maintenance treatment, or both treatments.
- Additional treatment often involves targeted treatment with a BTK inhibitor. Maintenance treatment often involves rituximab.
- If first-line treatment doesn't work or the lymphoma relapses, you may receive the same or a different type of treatment (second-line treatment).
- People with slow-growing MCL who have no symptoms usually don't get treatment. But they'll continue to be tested to detect any changes.

Questions to ask

- What is your experience as well as your team's experience with treating the type of lymphoma I have?
- Are my chances any better for one treatment than another? Less time-consuming? Less expensive?
- How will you know if the treatment is working?
- What are my options if the treatment stops working?
- What supportive care services are available to me during and after treatment?

share with us.

Take our survey and help make the NCCN Guidelines for Patients better for everyone!

NCCN.org/patients/comments

5

Treatment for early mantle cell lymphoma

Most people with mantle cell lymphoma (MCL) are diagnosed at a more advanced stage. But a small number of people have early-stage MCL. This chapter discusses how early MCL can be treated.

The early stages of mantle cell lymphoma (MCL) are stage 1 and stage 2.

Stage 1 MCL is defined as lymphoma in 1 lymph node or in 1 group of nearby lymph nodes.

Stage 2 MCL has affected 2 or more lymph nodes or groups of nearby lymph nodes.

Because these lymphomas occur in fewer areas in the body, people seldom show significant symptoms. That's one reason why MCL is rarely diagnosed at these stages.

Treatment for stage 1 and stage 2 MCL

Primary treatment

Radiation therapy, chemoimmunotherapy, or a combination of both can often control stage 1 or stage 2 MCL. Chemoimmunotherapy options for early MCL are listed in **Guide 5**.

In some cases, treatment for stage 1 or stage 2 MCL may not be needed right away. Instead, a watch-and-wait approach (also called active surveillance) is used to decide if or when to start treatment.

Guide 5
Primary drug treatments for early MCL (in alphabetical order)

Preferred treatments	**ABR**	Acalabrutinib, Bendamustine, plus Rituximab
	AR	Acalabrutinib plus Rituximab
	BR	Bendamustine plus Rituximab
Other recommended treatments	**CHOP plus Rituximab**	(Cyclophosphamide, Doxorubicin, Vincristine, Prednisone) plus Rituximab
	IR	Ibrutinib plus Rituximab
	LR	Lenalidomide plus Rituximab
	VR-CAP	(Bortezomib, Cyclophosphamide, Doxorubicin, Prednisone) plus Rituximab

People under active surveillance continue to have tests to keep an eye on their lymphoma. They see their doctor every 2 or 3 months, or longer if the disease has been stable for a while. If symptoms arise, they'll begin treatment.

Follow-up care

After primary treatment, your care team will evaluate your results to see how well the therapy worked. You may need additional treatment depending on your response to the primary treatment.

Complete response

If tests can no longer detect lymphoma, you've had a **complete response** to primary therapy. A complete response is often called remission.

The lymphoma may still return later, but a complete response may allow you to stop treatment and receive active surveillance. (If so, take time to enjoy the moment.)

Active surveillance means you'll continue to see your care team for follow-up tests, but you won't receive treatment. These tests look for signs that the lymphoma has returned.

Typical tests and schedules are:

- **Physical exam and lab tests** every 3 or 6 months for at least 5 years, then once a year or when recommended by your doctor
- **CT imaging** of your chest, abdomen, and pelvis no more than twice a year for the first 2 years if recommended by your doctor

If follow-up tests show that the lymphoma has relapsed, you'll need additional treatment.

Partial response

A **partial response** to primary therapy means that the lymphoma has decreased in size but is still there.

If you have a partial response, your doctor may recommend additional treatment to try to put the lymphoma into remission (complete response).

Progression

Progression means MCL has continued to grow or spread even with treatment. You'll need additional treatment to get the lymphoma under control.

Additional treatment

The choice of additional treatment depends on which treatment you had first. In general, if your earlier treatment was:

Only radiation therapy, then your additional treatment will likely be more aggressive. See *Chapter 4: Treatment for advanced MCL*.

Chemoimmunotherapy with or without radiation therapy, then you'll probably need more aggressive therapy—the kind recommended for relapsed or refractory MCL. See *Chapter 6: Treatment for recurrent MCL*. In certain cases, though, relapsed MCL can be treated with the same type of therapy recommended for advanced-stage MCL. For such cases, see *Chapter 4: Treatment for advanced mantle cell lymphoma*.

Key points

- Early-stage mantle cell lymphoma (MCL) is found in fewer areas in the body. MCL is rarely diagnosed in its early stages.
- Radiation therapy or less intense chemoimmunotherapy may be enough to control lymphoma growth in early-stage MCL. Some people have both therapies.
- Some people with early-stage MCL may not need treatment immediately, depending on their age and health. Their doctors may choose to watch them instead.
- If symptoms begin, people with early MCL are re-evaluated. If necessary, they'll begin treatment with radiation therapy, chemoimmunotherapy, or both therapies.
- Early-stage MCL that completely responds to treatment (remission) may still relapse later on.
- Early-stage MCL that partially responds to less intense treatment will need more aggressive treatment.
- Early-stage MCL that continues to grow or spread after treatment will need the kind of treatment recommended for relapsed or refractory MCL.

Questions to ask

- How long do I have to decide about treatment, and is there a social worker or someone who can help me decide?
- Am I eligible for watch-and-wait?
- Do I have a choice of when to begin treatment? Can I choose the days and times of treatment?
- What follow-up care is needed after treatment?
- What are the chances of the lymphoma worsening or returning?

6

Treatment for recurrent mantle cell lymphoma

If first-line treatment doesn't work or the lymphoma returns or gets worse, other types of treatment are available. In addition to a number of effective, approved therapies, you can also look for a clinical trial that's recruiting patients with mantle cell lymphoma (MCL) like yours.

Recurrent mantle cell lymphoma (MCL) means the lymphoma hasn't gone away or has come back.

Recurrent MCL includes relapsed, refractory, and progressive MCL.

- **Relapsed** – A relapse is when MCL improves with treatment, but then eventually comes back.
- **Refractory** – Refractory disease is when treatment has no effect or the lymphoma worsens while you're on treatment. Refractory means MCL isn't responding to therapy.
- **Progressive** – Progressive lymphoma continues to grow or worsen after treatment.

MCL that has relapsed, is refractory, or is progressing after first-line therapy can be treated with another (second-line) therapy.

Second-line therapy

As with first-line therapy, the goal of second-line therapy is to achieve remission. Remission is when the signs and symptoms of lymphoma have disappeared.

The idea behind second-line treatment is to try a different strategy than first-line treatment. Treatment choices for relapsed, refractory, and progressive MCL are affected by your previous therapy, age, overall health, and other diseases or conditions you may have.

"Just look around you. Sometimes it's easy to forget that you are surrounded by people who care about your well-being and success!"

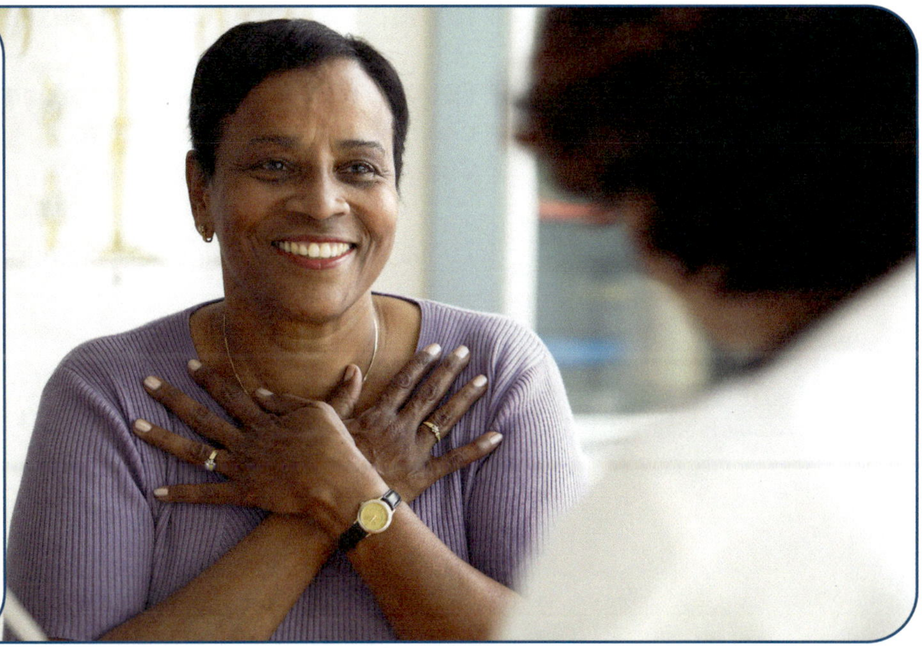

Preferred treatments for relapsed or refractory MCL

In recent years, clinical trials have shown that targeted therapy with one of the BTK inhibitors can be more effective than other therapies for relapsed or refractory MCL (if you didn't have a BTK inhibitor as first-line therapy). So the preferred second-line therapy includes a BTK inhibitor, either acalabrutinib (Calquence) or zanubrutinib (Brukinsa). See **Guide 6**.

If you've been prescribed one of these BTK inhibitors for second-line therapy, you may need to continue taking it indefinitely or until MCL relapses again.

Guide 6
Second-line therapies for relapsed or refractory MCL (in alphabetical order)

Preferred treatments	Acalabrutinib
	Lenalidomide plus Rituximab
	Zanubrutinib
Other recommended treatment	Ibrutinib with or without Rituximab
Treatments used in certain cases	Bendamustine plus Rituximab • Not recommended if you've been treated with Bendamustine before
	Bortezomib with or without Rituximab
	DHA (Dexamethasone, Cytarabine) and platinum-based chemotherapy plus Rituximab • Rituximab may be omitted if you've been treated with it before
	GEMOX (Gemcitabine, Oxaliplatin) plus Rituximab
	Ibrutinib and Venetoclax
	RBAC (Bendamustine, Low-Dose Cytarabine) plus Rituximab • Not recommended if you've been treated with Bendamustine before
	Venetoclax with or without Rituximab

Another preferred second-line therapy is a combination of lenalidomide (Revlimid) and rituximab (Rituxan).

Treatments used in certain cases of relapsed or refractory MCL

Other drug combinations are useful in specific cases of relapsed or refractory MCL. Options for second-line therapies used in certain cases are listed in the lower half of **Guide 6**.

Treatments for progressive MCL

If you've previously had one of the usual BTK inhibitors—acalabrutinib, ibrutinib, or zanubrutinib—but the lymphoma is progressing, you have a few options for second-line or subsequent therapy.

The simplest option may be trying a different BTK inhibitor called pirtobrutinib (Jaypirca). See **Guide 7**.

Additional treatment

If second-line therapy appears to be working (a complete response), then you may continue this treatment for as long as it keeps MCL under control.

You might also have additional treatment that may get the lymphoma under even better control.

The type of additional treatment you receive is based on several factors. An important factor is how well second-line therapy treated the lymphoma. Other factors include your age, overall health, and which treatments you've already had.

Additional treatments may include those that you haven't had yet: an allogeneic stem cell transplant with or without radiation therapy, high-dose chemotherapy and autologous stem cell transplant (HDT/ASCR), or active surveillance.

Guide 7
Therapies for progressive MCL, if you've already had a BTK inhibitor
(in alphabetical order)

Other BTK inhibitor	Pirtobrutinib
CAR T-cell therapy	Brexucabtagene autoleucel
	Lisocabtagene maraleucel
Bispecific antibody	Glofitamab-gxbm
	Mosunetuzumab-axgb and Polatuzumab vedotin-piiq

If you've had a partial response to second-line therapy, your additional therapy may include a bispecific antibody, CAR T-cell therapy, a different BTK inhibitor (pirtobrutinib), or active surveillance.

If the lymphoma doesn't respond or it progresses after second-line therapy, additional therapy may include CAR T-cell therapy, a different BTK inhibitor (pirtobrutinib), a bispecific antibody, a clinical trial, or having a different second-line therapy you haven't already had.

Follow-up care

After second-line treatment, you'll need to see your doctor and care team frequently so they can check how you're doing. You'll likely have follow-up visits every 3 to 6 months or as often as your care team recommends.

Follow-up tests often include in-person check-ups to evaluate how you feel, as well as evaluations such as a physical exam, blood tests, and imaging tests (CT scans). The follow-up plan is adapted for each person and can be adjusted for someone who's in a long remission (for example, less frequent follow-up visits).

Third-line and further therapies

Third-line therapy or further therapies for relapsed or refractory MCL generally include any treatment for MCL that you haven't already had.

Other recommended third-line and further therapies include:

- CAR T-cell therapy, if you haven't had it before
- Other BTK inhibitor (pirtobrutinib), if you haven't had it before
- Sonrotoclax (Beqalzi), a BCL-2 inhibitor, if you've had a BTK inhibitor before
- Clinical trial
- Low-dose radiation therapy for pain symptoms
- Additional supportive care

NCCN experts strongly encourage people with relapsed, refractory, or progressive MCL to ask their health care team how to find a relevant clinical trial.

Of course, you can ask for supportive care at any time to help relieve your lymphoma symptoms and reduce the side effects of treatment.

Supportive care

Supportive care is an important part of cancer care. The goal is to improve your quality of life during and after cancer treatment. Supportive care is for everyone with cancer and their families, not just for those at the end of life.

Supportive care includes a wide range of services. Supportive care prevents or manages the symptoms of cancer and the side effects of cancer treatment, like pain and cancer-related fatigue.

For people with relapsed, refractory, or progressive MCL, an important type of supportive care can be radiation therapy to relieve pain. Low-dose radiation therapy is not given to cure the lymphoma but to alleviate symptoms such as bone pain.

There's also treatment available for mouth sores and swelling (oral mucositis), which is a side effect of some lymphoma therapies.

Supportive care also addresses the mental, social, emotional, and spiritual concerns faced by people with cancer.

Supportive care provides help with additional needs, such as:

- Making treatment decisions
- Coordinating your care
- Paying for care
- Planning for advance care and end of life

Read more about the types of support you may receive in *NCCN Guidelines for Patients: Palliative Care*, available at NCCN.org/patientguidelines and on the NCCN Patient Guides for Cancer app.

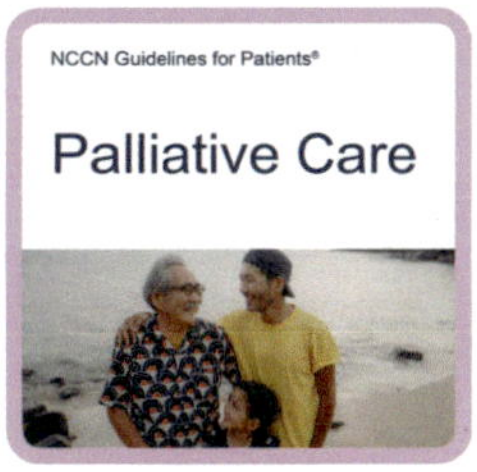

Advance care planning

Advance care planning is for anyone with lymphoma, not only for those who are very sick. Even when lymphoma is curable, talking about future scenarios should begin when treatment begins.

Advance care planning means deciding what care you would want if you become unable to make medical decisions for yourself. It's about making sure that your wishes are understood and respected.

You can decide if there's a point where you might want to stop lymphoma treatment. You can also decide what treatments you would want for symptom relief.

You can speak to your care team to set up an advance care plan early on, so you'll feel less stressed and better able to cope with your condition.

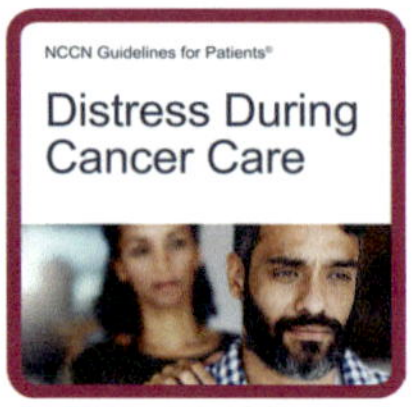

It's important to ask for help

Depression, anxiety, fear, and distress are very common feelings for people with lymphoma. These feelings can make it harder to deal with lymphoma and its treatment. They can hold you back even when you want to move forward.

Getting help when you're feeling worried or hopeless is an important part of lymphoma care. If you're feeling anxious or overwhelmed, ask your treatment team for help.

More information about cancer and distress is available at NCCN.org/patientguidelines and on the NCCN Patient Guides for Cancer app.

Key points

- If first-line therapy doesn't work or the lymphoma relapses, you can have second-line therapy that uses a different strategy.
- A preferred option for second-line therapy is a BTK inhibitor (if you didn't have one as a first-line therapy).
- NCCN experts strongly encourage people with relapsed, refractory, or progressive MCL to try to find a relevant clinical trial.
- You may have additional treatment after second-line therapy to get the lymphoma under control.
- Additional treatment, if appropriate, may include a different type of BTK inhibitor, CAR T-cell therapy, or another type of therapy you haven't had before.
- Supportive care is an important part of your treatment care. It can help prevent or reduce the side effects of treatment, among other things.
- Supportive care and advance care planning aren't just for those who are very sick or at the end of life, but for anyone with lymphoma and their loved ones.

Questions to ask

- Does this hospital or cancer center offer the best treatment for my lymphoma?
- Are there any programs to help pay for treatment?
- What should I know if I need to travel for treatment?
- Who should I contact with questions or concerns during weekends or non-office hours?
- Do you recommend that I consider a clinical trial for treatment?

"There's more hope now than there ever was. So don't give up. When hope is in the equation, the odds don't matter."

We want your feedback!

Our goal is to provide helpful and easy-to-understand information on cancer. Take our survey to let us know what we got right and what we could do better.
NCCN.org/patients/feedback

7
Other resources

Want to learn more? Here's how you can get additional help.

What else to know

This guide helps you know your options so you can make informed decisions and improve your cancer care. But it's not the only resource that you have.

Ask for as much information and help as you need. Many people are interested in learning more about:

- The details of their health and treatment
- Finding a health care practitioner who's experienced in lymphomas
- The side effects of lymphoma treatment
- How to get a second opinion
- The chances for lymphoma recurrence
- Getting financial help

What else to do

Your health care center can help you with next steps. It often has on-site resources to help meet your needs and find answers to your questions. Health care centers can also inform you of resources in your community.

In addition to help from your providers, the resources listed in the next section provide support for many people like yourself.

Where to get help

Look through the list below and visit the provided websites to learn more about these organizations.

Blood & Marrow Transplant Information Network (BMT InfoNet)
bmtinfonet.org

Blood Cancer United
bloodcancerunited.org

Cancer*Care*
cancercare.org

Imerman Angels
imermanangels.org

GRACE
cancergrace.org

Lymphoma Research Foundation
lymphoma.org

Mantle Cell Lymphoma Alliance
mantlecellalliance.org

National Bone Marrow Transplant Link (nbmtLINK)
nbmtlink.org

NMDP
nmdp.org

PAN Foundation
panfoundation.org

Stupid Cancer
stupidcancer.org

Triage Cancer
triagecancer.org

Questions to ask

- Who can I talk to about help with housing, food, and other basic needs?
- What help is available for transportation, childcare, and home care?
- What other services are available to me and my caregivers?
- How can I connect with others and build a support system?
- Who can I talk to if I don't feel safe at home, at work, or in my neighborhood?

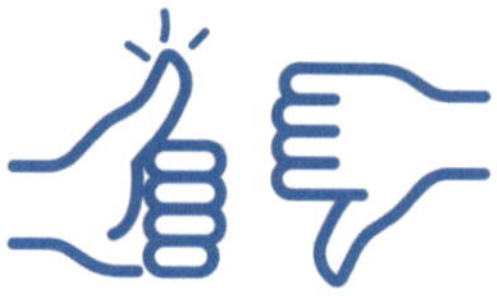

Let us know what you think!

Please take a moment to complete an online survey about the NCCN Guidelines for Patients.
NCCN.org/patients/response

Words to know

active surveillance
A period of testing for changes in cancer status while not receiving treatment.

additional treatment
A shorter, more intense treatment phase to further reduce the number of lymphoma cells after primary treatment.

allogeneic stem cell transplant
A cancer treatment that replaces abnormal blood stem cells with healthy donor stem cells. These stem cells create a new immune system to wipe out any lymphoma cells left behind after previous therapy.

autologous stem cell transplant
A cancer treatment that removes a patient's own healthy stem cells and later returns them to the bone marrow after chemotherapy. Also called high-dose chemotherapy with autologous stem cell rescue (HDT/ASCR).

B cell
A type of white blood cell (lymphocyte) that protects the body from infection. Also called B lymphocyte.

biopsy
A procedure that removes fluid or tissue samples to be tested for disease.

bispecific antibody
A targeted therapy that binds to 2 different targets at the same time.

bone marrow
The sponge-like tissue in the center of most bones where new blood cells are made.

bone marrow aspiration
A procedure that removes a liquid bone marrow sample to test for a disease.

bone marrow biopsy
A procedure that removes bone and solid bone marrow samples to test for a disease.

B symptoms
Fevers, heavy sweats, and unexpected weight loss caused by B-cell lymphomas.

BTK inhibitor
A drug that blocks an enzyme called BTK. Blocking BTK slows or stops cancer cells from growing.

cancer stage
A rating of cancer based on its location and extent.

CAR T-cell therapy
An immunotherapy that alters a person's own T cells to recognize and destroy their cancer.

chemotherapy
Cancer drugs that stop the cell life cycle so cells don't increase in number.

chromosomes
Structures within cells that contain coded instructions for cell function.

clinical trial
A type of research that assesses how well health tests or treatments work in people.

complete blood count (CBC)
A lab test that measures the number of red blood cells, white blood cells, and platelets.

complete blood count (CBC) with differential
A lab test that measures the number of blood cells including each type of white blood cell.

complete response
An absence of all signs and symptoms of cancer after treatment.

computed tomography (CT)
A test that uses x-rays from many angles to make a picture of the insides of the body.

diagnosis
An identification of an illness based on tests.

early stage
A cancer that has had little or no growth into nearby tissues.

echocardiogram
A test that uses sound waves to make pictures of the heart.

gastrointestinal (GI) tract
The group of organs through which food passes after being eaten. Also called the digestive tract.

gene
Coded instructions for making proteins that control how cells behave and make new cells.

hematopathologist
A doctor who examines cancers of the blood and immune cells.

imaging
A test that makes pictures (images) of the insides of the body.

immune system
The body's natural defense against disease.

immunomodulator
A cancer drug that modifies some parts of the body's disease-fighting system.

immunotherapy
A treatment with drugs that help the body find and destroy cancer cells.

involved-site radiation therapy (ISRT)
Treatment with radiation that's focused on areas of cancer growth.

lactate dehydrogenase (LDH) test
A blood test that indicates the amount of lymphoma and cellular damage in the body.

lumbar puncture
A procedure that removes spinal fluid with a needle. Also called a spinal tap.

lymph
A clear fluid containing white blood cells.

lymph node
A small, bean-shaped, disease-fighting structure.

lymphadenopathy
A medical term meaning swollen lymph nodes.

lymphatic system
A network of organs and vessels that collects and transports lymph fluid.

lymphocyte
One of three main types of white blood cells that help protect the body from infections.

lymphoma
A cancer of white blood cells (lymphocytes) within the lymphatic system.

maintenance treatment
A treatment phase given to prolong good treatment results.

mantle zone
A ring of B cells that surrounds the germinal center of a follicle inside lymph nodes.

primary treatment
The first treatment that is given to greatly reduce the extent of cancer.

prognosis
The likely course and outcome of a disease.

progression
The growth or spread of cancer after being tested or treated.

radiation therapy
A treatment that uses intense energy to kill cancer cells.

refractory cancer
Cancer that doesn't respond to treatment.

relapse
The return of cancer after a period of improvement.

side effect
An unhealthy or unpleasant physical or emotional response to treatment.

supportive care
Health care that includes symptom relief and improving quality of life. Also called palliative care.

T cell
A type of white blood cell (lymphocyte) that attacks infected cells and cancer cells.

targeted therapy
A drug treatment that targets specific molecules that keep cancer cells alive and growing.

translocation
The switching of parts between chromosomes.

uric acid
A chemical that is released into the blood when cells and other substances in the body break down.

white blood cell
A type of blood cell that fights disease and infection

NCCN Contributors

This patient guide is based on the NCCN Clinical Practice Guidelines in Oncology (NCCN Guidelines®) for B-Cell Lymphomas, Version 4.2026. It was adapted, reviewed, and published with help from the following people:

Dorothy A. Shead, MS
Senior Director
Patient Information Operations

John Murphy
Senior Medical Writer

Lisa Diehl
Production Layout Artist

The NCCN Clinical Practice Guidelines in Oncology (NCCN Guidelines®) for B-Cell Lymphomas, Version 4.2026, were developed by the following NCCN Panel Members:

Andrew D. Zelenetz, MD, PhD/Chair
Memorial Sloan Kettering Cancer Center

Leo I. Gordon, MD/Vice Chair
Robert H. Lurie Comprehensive Cancer Center of Northwestern University

Jeremy S. Abramson, MD, MMSc
Mass General Cancer Center

Ranjana H. Advani, MD
Stanford Cancer Institute

Alaa Altahan, MD
St. Jude Children's Research Hospital/ The University of Tennessee Health Science Center

Babis Andreadis, MD, MSCE
UCSF Helen Diller Family Comprehensive Cancer Center

Nancy L. Bartlett, MD
Siteman Cancer Center at Barnes-Jewish Hospital and Washington University School of Medicine

L. Elizabeth Budde, MD, PhD
City of Hope National Medical Center

Paolo F. Caimi, MD
Case Comprehensive Cancer Center/ University Hospitals Seidman Cancer Center and Cleveland Clinic Taussig Cancer Institute

Sven DeVos, MD, PhD
UCLA Jonsson Comprehensive Cancer Center

Bhagirathbhai Dholaria, MD
Vanderbilt-Ingram Cancer Center

Luis E. Fayad, MD
The University of Texas MD Anderson Cancer Center

Sameh Gaballa, MD
Moffitt Cancer Center

Thomas M. Habermann, MD
Mayo Clinic Comprehensive Cancer Center

Francisco Hernandez-Ilizaliturri, MD
Roswell Park Comprehensive Cancer Center

Boyu Hu, MD
Huntsman Cancer Institute at the University of Utah

Manali Kamdar, MD
University of Colorado Cancer Center

Yasmin Karimi, MD
University of Michigan Rogel Cancer Center

Christopher R. Kelsey, MD
Duke Cancer Institute

Rebecca King, MD
Mayo Clinic Comprehensive Cancer Center

Justin Kline, MD
The UChicago Medicine Comprehensive Cancer Center

Susan Krivacic, MPAff
Patient advocate

*Ann S. LaCasce, MD, MMSc
Dana-Farber/Brigham and Women's Cancer Center

Daniel Landsburg, MD
Abramson Cancer Center at the University of Pennsylvania

Megan Lim, MD, PhD
Memorial Sloan Kettering Cancer Center

Marcus Messmer, MD
Fox Chase Cancer Center

Priyanka Pophali, MD
University of Wisconsin Carbone Cancer Center

Rachel Rabinovitch, MD
University of Colorado Cancer Center

Praveen Ramakrishnan, MD, MS
UT Southwestern Simmons Comprehensive Cancer Center

Erin Reid, MD
UC San Diego Moores Cancer Center

Peter Riedell, MD
The UChicago Medicine Comprehensive Cancer Center

Kenneth B. Roberts, MD
Yale Cancer Center/Smilow Cancer Hospital

Aditi Saha, MD
O'Neal Comprehensive Cancer Center at UAB

Naoyuki G. Saito, MD, PhD
Indiana University Melvin and Bren Simon Comprehensive Cancer Center

Yazeed Sawalha, MD
The Ohio State University Comprehensive Cancer Center - James Cancer Hospital and Solove Research Institute

*Stephen D. Smith, MD
Fred Hutchinson Cancer Center

Lode J. Swinnen, MBChB, MD
Johns Hopkins Kimmel Cancer Center

Joseph Tuscano, MD
UC Davis Comprehensive Cancer Center

*Julie M. Vose, MD, MBA
Fred & Pamela Buffett Cancer Center

NCCN

Mary Dwyer, MS
Senior Director, Guidelines Operations

Hema Sundar, PhD
Senior Manager, Global Clinical Content

* Reviewed this patient guide. For disclosures, visit NCCN.org/disclosures.

NCCN Cancer Centers

For contact information, visit NCCN.org/cancercenters.

Abramson Cancer Center
at the University of Pennsylvania
Philadelphia, Pennsylvania

Case Comprehensive Cancer Center/
University Hospitals Seidman Cancer Center and
Cleveland Clinic Taussig Cancer Institute
Cleveland, Ohio

City of Hope National Medical Center
Duarte, California

Dana-Farber Cancer Institute
Boston, Massachusetts

Duke Cancer Institute
Durham, North Carolina

Fox Chase Cancer Center
Philadelphia, Pennsylvania

Fred & Pamela Buffett Cancer Center
Omaha, Nebraska

Fred Hutchinson Cancer Center
Seattle, Washington

Huntsman Cancer Institute at the University of Utah
Salt Lake City, Utah

Indiana University Melvin and Bren Simon
Comprehensive Cancer Center
Indianapolis, Indiana

Johns Hopkins Kimmel Cancer Center
Baltimore, Maryland

Mass General Brigham Cancer Institute
Boston, Massachusetts

Mayo Clinic Comprehensive Cancer Center
Phoenix/Scottsdale, Arizona
Jacksonville, Florida
Rochester, Minnesota

Memorial Sloan Kettering Cancer Center
New York, New York

Moffitt Cancer Center
Tampa, Florida

O'Neal Comprehensive Cancer Center at UAB
Birmingham, Alabama

Robert H. Lurie Comprehensive Cancer Center
of Northwestern University
Chicago, Illinois

Roswell Park Comprehensive Cancer Center
Buffalo, New York

Siteman Cancer Center at Barnes-Jewish Hospital
and WashU Medicine
St. Louis, Missouri

St. Jude Children's Research Hospital/
The University of Tennessee Health Science Center
Memphis, Tennessee

Stanford Cancer Institute
Stanford, California

The Ohio State University Comprehensive Cancer Center -
James Cancer Hospital and Solove Research Institute
Columbus, Ohio

The UChicago Medicine Comprehensive Cancer Center
Chicago, Illinois

The University of Texas MD Anderson Cancer Center
Houston, Texas

UC Davis Comprehensive Cancer Center
Sacramento, California

UC San Diego Moores Cancer Center
La Jolla, California

UCLA Jonsson Comprehensive Cancer Center
Los Angeles, California

UCSF Helen Diller Family Comprehensive Cancer Center
San Francisco, California

University of Colorado Cancer Center
Aurora, Colorado

University of Michigan Rogel Cancer Center
Ann Arbor, Michigan

University of Wisconsin Carbone Cancer Center
Madison, Wisconsin

UT Southwestern Simmons
Comprehensive Cancer Center
Dallas, Texas

Vanderbilt-Ingram Cancer Center
Nashville, Tennessee

Yale Cancer Center/Smilow Cancer Hospital
New Haven, Connecticut

Notes

Index

Made in the USA
Monee, IL
05 November 2026

67386681R00038